DIABET
TYPE 2
GROCERY
AND FOODS
LIST

By : Jason Manson

Disclaimer :

The information contained in this book should be used aa a reference only, and it is not intended to give any medical advice.

Important notice

The data and values in this book are pulled from USDA data center and CDC, these data are subject to further updates, and we are constantly improving this book to keep it relevant and practical.

To get in touch with us, or to join our community of 873 type 2 diabetes patients and benefit from support, and free resources, please email us at.

latcarl3@gmail.com

Table of Contents

I. How to use this list

▪ I.1 Nutrition notes for diabetes:

· Carbs:

Carbohydrates (carbs) are a type of sugar found in natural and processed foods, these carbs are the ones that affect directedly the sugar level in your blood, there are carbs that spike the sugar level in your blood quickly, these foods are called "high glycemic index foods", meanwhile, other foods will take a longer time to increase the sugar level in your blood, these foods are called "low glycemic index foods).

To keep diabetes under control, you should know how much carbs you take throughout the day, according to CDC (the US centers for disease control and prevention), a diabetic person should aim for 200-250 grams of carbs a day or 45 to 60 grams of carbohydrates per meal, this quantity may (and should) be adjusted according to the age, weight, health, activity, and whether the person is taking insulin injections or not, so we recommend to discuss with your doctor the amount of carbs you should not exceed for each day.

This list is intended to help type 2 diabetes to make better choices about their food.

- **Calories :**

Controlling calories intake is important for diabetes type 2 to lose extra weight and maintain a healthy one, typically, as a diabetes patient, you should limit calories intake to 1500-1800 per day.

In this list, We added the calorie content of foods to help you better control them.

- **Fibers:**

Eating fibers is the greatest and the easiest way to control blood glycemic levels, that's why we added the fiber content for each food in this list.

- **I.2 How to use the list:**

Use this list as you use a dictionary to look up foods

For each food, you will find its content in carbs, calories, fat, and fibers.

There is also an important column in this list: **"Comment"**, in this column, you will know whether to **avoid the food**, **eat it in**

moderation, or **eat it as much as you want**, please see the following extract from the list:

Food	Measure	Calories	Fat (g)	Fiber (g)	Carbs (g)	Comment
Acesulfame potassium	1/2 gram	0	0	0	0.5	Eat as much as you want
Adzuki beans	1 cup	329	0.5	25	124	Limit to 2 cups a day
Agave	1 tbsp	21	0.5	na	76	Eat in moderation (do not exceed 3 times per day)

- **Remark:**

when **"eat as much as you want"** is mentionned for a food, it means that the food will not spike your blood sugar whatever the quantity you eat, however, you have to keep an eye over the calories you take in order to keep a healthy weight, that's why, never overeate a food even if "eat as much as you want" is mentionned.

Remeber that the golden Word for diabetes is " Moderation"

Visit us :

www.diabetes2.club

we launched the diabetes2.club website to help you better manage type 2 diabetes in the easiest way.

You can visit us to get free printable check lists, sheets, lists, and notes about food planning, nutrition, tracking, and other day to day important material for type 2 diabetes.

II. How do we qualify the foods in this list:

All nutrition data in this list are coming from the nutrition data available in the database of the USDA (U.S. Department of Agriculture), so, the nutrition information in this list is trustworthy.

Our method to qualify the foods in this list (whether to eat food in moderation, avoid it, or eat it with no restriction) is based on two scientific facts:

1: The maximum carbs amount that a diabetic should not exceed is 250 g per day.

2: A healthy alimentation of a type 2 diabetic should contain carbs, protein, and non-starchy foods (please see the next section for more information about this subject)

III. How to do your grocery shopping

Grocery shopping is the starting point to controlling your blood sugar level.

The right planning of your grocery shopping on a weekly basis (preferably), buying fresh foods, avoiding as much as you can processed foods, and paying attention to food labels will help you to maintain a healthy life.

A good meal plan will include non-starchy vegetables like broccoli, spinach, and green bean..., fewer added sugars, less refined grains such as white bread, rice, and pasta, and more whole foods.
Non-starchy foods are foods that have low carbs and low calories, these foods will keep you full for a long time, they will give your body the vitamins and minerals that it needs, and will keep your blood sugar level low.
When you do your grocery, try to make 50% of your shopping cart composed of non-starchy foods, 25% from proteins like chicken, turkey, fish, eggs, and the remaining 25% from carb foods like fruits, pasta, and yogurt…

Here is a list of some of non-starchy foods:

Non-starchy food list:

Amaranth
Artichoke
Artichoke hearts
arugula,
Asparagus

Baby corn
Bamboo shoots
Bean sprouts
Beans (green, wax, Italian)
Beets
Broccoli
Brussels sprouts
Cabbage (green, bok choy, Chinese)
Carrots
Cauliflower
Celery
Chayote
chicory,
Cucumber
Daikon
Eggplant
endive,
escarole,
Greens (collard, kale, mustard, turnip)
Hearts of palm
Jicama
Kohlrabi
Leeks
lettuce,
Mushrooms
Okra
Onions
Pea pods
Peppers
radicchio,
Radishes
romaine,
Rutabaga
Salad greens

spinach,
Sprouts
Sugar snap peas
Swiss chard
Tomato
Turnips
Water chestnuts
watercress
Yard-long beans
zucchini

When you do grocery for processed and canned foods, then you should pay attention to the food label, especially look at their carbs content.

Make sure to verify also the processed foods labeled as **"Low sugar**" or as **"Low carbs foods** ", these foods may sound healthy, but in reality, they may contain high carbs content.

Here is how to read a food label :

1. Check the **Serving size** first. All the numbers on this label are for a 2/3-cup serving.
2. **This package has 8 servings.** If you eat the whole thing, you are eating 8 times the amount of calories, carbs, fat, etc., shown on the label.
3. **Total Carbohydrate** shows you types of carbs in the food, including sugar and fiber.
4. Choose foods with **more fiber, vitamins, and minerals.**
5. Choose foods with **lower calories, saturated fat, sodium, and added sugars.** Avoid *trans* fat.

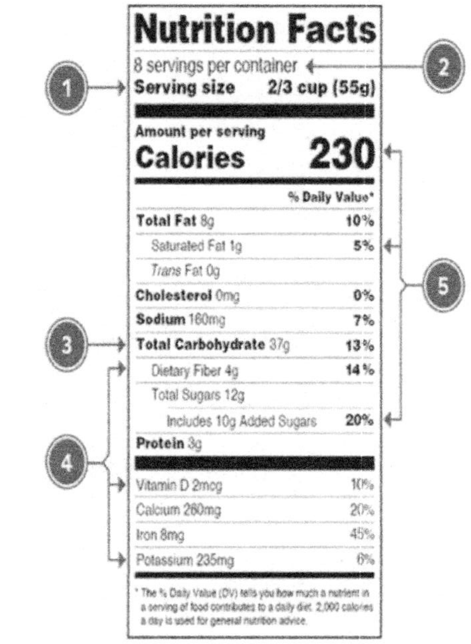

Source CDC.gov

Link:

https://www.cdc.gov/diabetes/managing/eat-well/food-labels.html

VI. Control your carbs intake: the Plate method

The plate method is the easiest way to control your carbs intake, you only need a 9 inches plate.

1. Take a 9-inch plate.
2. Fill it with foods as shown in the next figure

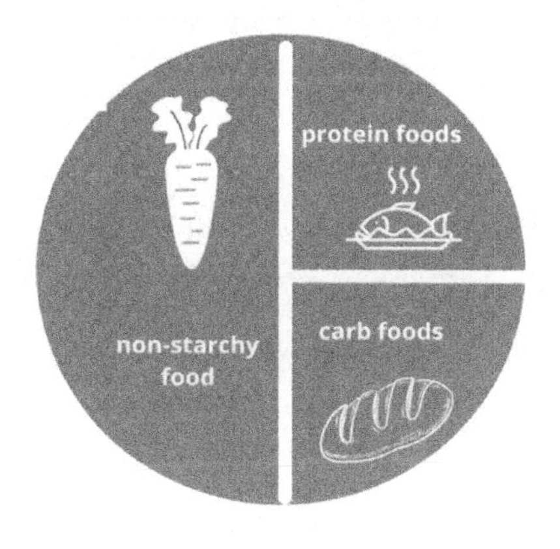

Half of your plate should be filled with non-starchy food.

1/4 of your plate should be filled with protein foods

And the remaining 1/4 should be filled with carb foods.

Here is an example of meal planning using this method:

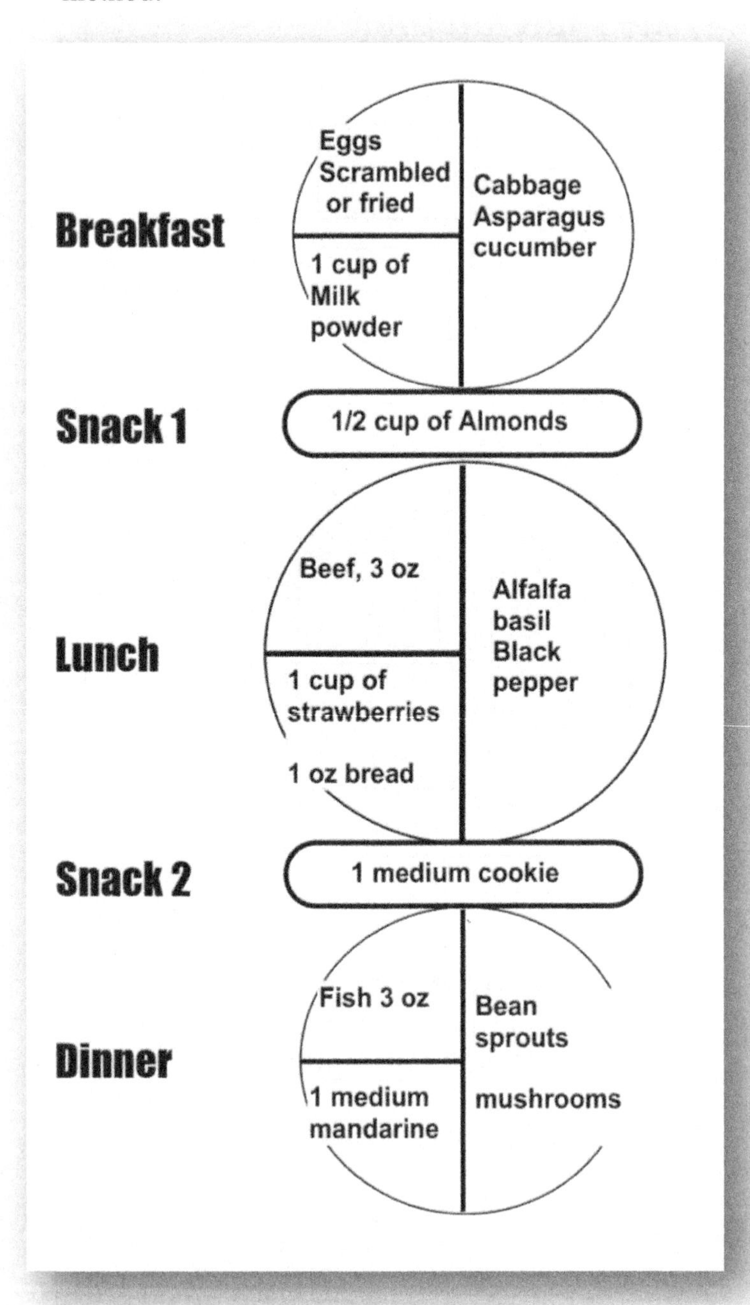

To get a blank printable plate planner to plan your meals, please visit our website and download it for free, or to get your ready to use diabetes type 2 meal planner.

Visit us on: www.diabetes2.club

V. Side note about tracking

If you have type 2 diabetes and are wondering how often you should perform your follow-up tests, know that there are several tests you can perform depending on your case:

- Daily: Through your portable meter, you can measure your blood glucose level directly and easily from home.
- At each medical consultation: a medical consultation is an excellent opportunity to measure your follow-up examination and to check the functioning of your organs.
- Every 3 months: take a blood test to measure your HbA1c, which is the blood sugar level in the past three months, and which should be less than 48mmol/mol
- At least once a year: consider having more in-depth tests to assess the functioning of organs that may be negatively affected by the disease: kidney function test, lipid test, cardiology test, eye and retina exam, dental exam, and foot exam.

V. FAQ about type 2 diabetes:

What is Type 2 Diabetes?

Considered as the most common among populations, Type 2 diabetes is a result of too high level of sugar (glucose) in the blood. Type 2 diabetes occurs when the insulin the pancreas makes can't operate properly or the pancreas is not able to make enough insulin. This leads to high blood glucose levels, so the body is not capable of using energy from food correctly.

Type 2 diabetes vs. Insulin resistance:

Type 2 diabetes is related to insulin resistance. When cells in the muscles, fat, and liver don't respond well to insulin, they can't easily take up glucose from the blood to use it for energy. In this case, the pancreas makes more insulin, and as a result of that, the blood sugar level gradually rises. However, over time, the pancreas produces less insulin, and the cells resist it. This also causes too much sugar in the blood.

Type 2 diabetes occurs most often in middle-aged or older people, but it can also affect kids and teenagers who suffer from overweight or obesity in early childhood.

What does Type 2 diabetes do to your body?

Type 2 diabetes can affect the everyday life of people who suffer from it. In the beginning, people with Type 2 Diabetes have symptoms like excessive thirst, need to urinate frequently during the day, unintentional weight loss, and fatigue.

It can also increase the risk of severe problems with the eyes like blurred vision, heart, and nerves.

Wounds may take a longer time to heal for people with Type 2 diabetes who can, unfortunately, experience genital itching or thrush. To pursue a normal life, people with Type 2 diabetes have to transform their diet, take long-term medicines, and go for regular check-ups.

The aggravating factors of the disease are mostly being overweight, inactivity, or heredity.

Why does Type 2 diabetes get you tired?

Fatigue is usually associated with Type 2 diabetes. Researchers have found that the main cause of tiredness is uncontrolled blood glucose.

If there is not enough insulin produced by the pancreas, or if the body is not responding to the insulin as it should be, the body will use fat to generate the energy it needs.

Energy is produced from the split of a molecule found in the body called ATP (adenosine triphosphate) into another molecule called ADP (Adenosine diphosphate).

After expelling one of its phosphates for energy, ATP turns to ADP, and, If there is no energy source available, the ATP cannot get back the phosphate it donates, and this is the chemical process that leads to physical fatigue.

Does Type 2 diabetes cause weight loss?

Unintentional weight loss can be a symptom of Type 2 diabetes. As a reminder, in the case of Type 2 diabetes, the insulin that transforms sugar or glucose into energy is either not enough produced by the pancreas or the body can't use it effectively. As a result, instead of being converted into energy, the rate of sugar rises in the blood.

When the body can't get the energy it needs, it starts burning fat and muscle for energy, as a consequence, there is weight loss.

Can Type 2 diabetes be cured?

Unfortunately, there is no cure for Type 2 diabetes. But even with the absence of a cure, people can reverse this chronic disease.

Through diet changes and weight loss, people with Type 2 diabetes can reach and maintain normal blood sugar levels without having to take any medication (at least in the beginning).

With diet and exercise, it is possible to have a normal life, without trouble controlling glucose, or any health problems related to diabetes.

Type 2 diabetes hyperglycemia, what is it? What are its symptoms and how to reverse it?

Type 2 diabetes hyperglycemia refers to high levels of sugar or glucose in the blood.

In general, a person has hyperglycemia when his blood glucose level is higher than 130 mg/dl before eating, and higher than 180 mg/dl after starting to eat a meal.

The main symptoms are frequent urge to urinate, excessive thirst, unusual hunger, headaches, blurred vision, weight loss, irritability, and fatigue.

These symptoms may not occur at once and take sometimes years to be noticeable. But they aggravate when blood sugar levels stay high. Treatment of type 2 diabetes includes controlling blood sugar levels and using medications or insulin if recommended.

Losing weight through diet and exercise also helps to maintain normal sugar levels in the blood, and help in reversing hyperglycemia.

Type 2 diabetes hypoglycemia, what is it? What are its symptoms and how to reverse it?

Hypoglycemia is the condition of having a very low sugar level in the blood, it occurs when the level of glucose in the blood falls below 72 mg/dl.

The symptoms of hypoglycemia can lead the person to sweat, fatigue, and feel dizzy. In severe and prolonged cases, hypoglycemia causes seizures or coma if not treated.

By controlling blood sugar levels, a person with Type 2 diabetes hypoglycemia can prevent this pathology.

A quick fix for hypoglycemia may be eating or drinking 15 to 20g of fast-acting carbohydrates like sweets, glucose tablets, or fruit juice before meals.

Type 2 diabetes control without medication:

At the beginning of Type 2 diabetes, the body usually produces a lot of insulin, unfortunately, the body can't use it efficiently. At this time, there is still no need for medication.

When the body stops making enough insulin, then the person with Type 2 diabetes may need medicine to manage the disease combined with a healthy diet, exercise, and weight loss.

How to control diabetes during pregnancy?

Diabetes is a chronic disease that women should watch carefully during months of pregnancy.

To stay safe, pregnant women must keep blood sugar at safe levels, and check regularely how the baby is growing.

In the first three months of pregnancy, women can take folic acid, which is the man-made version of vitamin folate, also known as vitamin B9, Folic acid helps the body produce healthy red blood cells.

During pregnancy, women should stop taking certain medications and do eye and kidneys check-ups. If she treats her diabetes with insulin, she needs to always have something sweet with her to prevent hypoglycemia. On the other hand, if sugar levels in the bloodstream are too high, she needs to see a doctor.

Why is it important to control diabetes?

The problems caused by diabetes are serious, the disease can affect almost every part of the body. Good control of diabetes during the first year can diminish the future risk of health complications.

When diabetes is not controlled, high blood sugar levels cause inflammation and changes at the cellular level, the body will then produces less insulin, and struggles to treat excess glucose in the bloodstream, which can lead to circulatory issues years later.

In the long-term, health problems occur, they are either microvascular related to eye disease, kidney disease, and poor circulation to the limbs, or macrovascular like heart disease and stroke.

How to control diabetes without losing weight?

Usually, people with diabetes need to maintain a healthy weight.

To avoid non-healthy weight loss while controlling diabetes, people need to have a special diet that is healthy and not restrictive at the same time. The key is to select nutrient-rich foods rather than sugary, and fatty foods.

These nutrient foods include nuts, seeds, avocado, nut butter, and coconut. Nutrient-dense carbohydrates like beans, quinoa, brown rice, and granola. This diet can also help people gain weight while keeping health benefits, and controlling blood sugar levels.

Control diabetes with fasting:

During the first hours of fasting, the body initially uses stored sources of glucose, and then later, it will break down body fat to use as it a source of energy.

Using the body's fat as energy can lead, in the long term, to weight loss, because of that, fasting diabetics need to consume more slowly absorbed foods (with low glycemic index) just before the first hours of fasting, these include fruits, vegetables, and salad. Diabetics need also to take their medication for good diabetes control.

However, fasting is forbidden for people who use insulin as a treatment for diabetes or the ones that have diabetes complications such as serious damage to the eyes, kidneys, or nerves in the hands and feet.

The risk of too low blood sugar levels after fasting (hypo) is high for people who take insulin. To prevent hypo, they have to test their blood glucose levels more often.

The opposite situation can happen if blood sugar levels become too high. This can cause diabetic ketoacidosis (DKA) which is life-threatening and requires hospital treatment. The symptoms of DKA are: feeling very thirsty and urinating a lot.

Diabetes control health outcomes:

When diabetes is well controlled, it is easier to reduce fatigue, bladder problems, and other symptoms of diabetes. Furthermore, managing diabetes well can diminish vision problems, dementia, and other severe medical issues. People who control their diabetes can also expect the same longevity as people without medical conditions.

On the other hand, out-of-control blood sugar levels can lead to hypoglycemia or diabetic ketoacidosis. In the long term, if diabetes stays uncontrolled, important organs can be damaged like the heart, kidneys, eyes, and nerves, but when diabetes is well managed through diet, exercise and medication, diabetics can avoid the most debilitating conditions.

Diabetes hunger control:

If glucose doesn't get into the cells when needed, diabetes can cause hunger.

To avoid hunger or food cravings, diabetics should eat regularly, especially in breakfast, and incorporate proteins into the meals. Some people's low-sugar hunger continues even with eating, in this case, taking insulin or insulin-sensitizing medication could be needed, but overeating can lead to spikes in blood sugar and weight gain.

The good news is that hunger decreases with better blood sugar control by eating more vegetables, fruits, and non-starchy foods.

Diabetes control in the elderly:

Diabetes requires careful treatment, especially in older people.

Through meal plan changes, exercise, and medication plans, people with diabetes can live longer and healthier. Here are the main actions to follow in order to keep a good sugar level.

First of all, older people like all people with diabetes should eat healthy food with a low glycemic index including sugar from fruit. Creating a healthy meal plan with a dietitian can help them follow a suitable diet.

Exercising for 30 minutes a day 5 days a week, walking, swimming, and cycling help people control their glucose level, manage their weight, and stay strong. Strength training like free weights, resistance bands or yoga builds muscle and helps control glucose levels.

Checking glucose levels regularly is also very important for older people. The main reason is that they have a higher risk of hypoglycemia when taking diabetes medications.

Another important thing is to never miss a dose of medication. A variety of ways exist to organize a person's medicines: pillboxes, alarms, computers, watches, and smartphones as a reminder to take medication.

To reduce the risk of heart disease and stroke, older people have to get blood pressure and cholesterol levels checked regularly.

Last but not least, feet have to be examined every day for cuts or signs of infection. Feet should be clean, lotions need to be used to avoid dryness, and shoes must be comfortable to avoid blisters.

Diabetes control tips:

To control diabetes, few changes in lifestyle are needed. Among the common tips, regular physical activity helps people with diabetes feel better, and it also improves sensitivity to insulin, as a consequence, blood sugar levels can become more stable.

Activities like aerobics, walking or jogging, and resistance exercises like working out with weights, and stretching are beneficial. In fact, exercising lowers blood sugar.

Regarding foods, a well-balanced diet with non-starchy vegetables, berries, citrus fruits, fish, poultry, non-dairy fat products, lean meat… some vegetarian protein like tofu, cereals with whole grain, like quinoa, brown rice, whole oats, and whole wheat… is recommended.

People with diabetes should also eat three healthy meals a day spaced out with the same amount of carbs, and avoid processed food (because of their high glycemic index). On the other hand, stress can cause high blood sugar and makes the body less sensitive to insulin. Studies showed that people with type 1 diabetes found that their blood sugar levels go up under mental stress, also people with type 2 diabetes who are under pressure see their glucose go up.

To relax, stressed people can spend time with friends, meditate, have positive thoughts, avoid negative ones and get therapy if possible. If diabetics are smoking, quitting the bad habit gives better control of blood sugar levels.

Finally, they must drastically reduce alcohol consumption because it increases hypoglycemia risks for people under insulin treatment or diabetes medication.

Diabetes control with vegetables

Non-starchy vegetables are one of the most suitable foods for people with diabetes. They are full of essential vitamins, and minerals that help regulate blood sugar.

Thanks to their very low amounts of sugar and high levels of fiber, people with diabetes can eat as many as they want of non-starchy vegetables without worrying about high blood sugar spikes.

These vegetables include artichokes, asparagus, avocados, broccoli, cabbage, cauliflower, celery, cucumbers, onions, tomatoes, squashes, and zucchini…

Leafy greens are also considered as non-starchy vegetables, they are full-packed of nutrients.

Some of the best leafy greens to incorporate into a diabetes diet are spinach and kale thanks to their high level of vitamin C. This vitamin helps manage diabetes in people with Type 2 diabetes.

They also contain specific antioxidants that help eyes from complications. In addition to vegetables, natural fat like extra-virgin olive oil reduces the risk of heart disease and contains strong antioxidants. These antioxidants help reduce inflammation, protect cells, and decrease blood pressure.

Last but not least, apple cider vinegar helps to improve insulin sensitivity, lowers fasting blood sugar levels, and reduces blood sugar response by 20% when paired with meals rich in carbs.

Diabetes control with vitamins:

There are many types of vitamins and supplements that can be helpful for people with Type 2 diabetes, however, these supplements can never replace diabetes treatment, and this is why it is always important to consult a doctor before taking any vitamin or supplement.

Here are some examples of vitamins and supplements that are good for diabetics:

Cinnamon, in whole form or extract, helps lower blood glucose levels. It can also help treat diabetes.

On the other hand, chromium, used in the metabolism of carbohydrates, is safe for most people, but there is a risk that chromium might lower blood sugar levels and damage the kidney at high doses.

Another vitamin is Benfotiamine, which is a supplemental form of thiamine. This lipid-soluble can penetrate cell membranes and prevent some diabetic complications.

To reduce pain from diabetic neuropathy (dysfunction in one or more nerves), Alpha-lipoic acid (ALA) injections improve symptoms of neuropathy in the short term, it can reduce oxidative stress, lower fasting blood sugar levels, and decrease insulin resistance.

Moreover, Magnesium which is an essential nutrient helps regulate blood pressure and insulin sensitivity. A high magnesium diet may also reduce the risk of diabetes.

Finally, green tea -an essential drink- contains polyphenols, which are antioxidants, Epigallocatechin gallate (EGCG), the main antioxidant of green tea may have numerous health benefits including lower cardiovascular disease risk, prevention of type 2 diabetes, improved glucose control, and better insulin activity.

Manage Diabetes without Medication:

Diabetes may not need medications at least at the beginning, they should try to take make healthy lifestyle changes to better manage the disease.

First of all, eating healthy nutrition with low carbohydrates, fruits and vegetables, whole grains, lean proteins, healthy fat, and high-quality proteins is the first step. Furthermore, losing 10% of weight can help control blood sugar; reduce cholesterol levels, lower blood pressure, and risk of complications.

No one can argue about the effects of exercising regularly (30 minutes a day walking, biking, or running) in the decrease of blood sugar levels, and increasing insulin resistance. It will also help regulate blood pressure and cholesterol levels.

By testing their blood sugar level regularly, diabetics can see the patterns and take actions to lower their blood sugar levels. Moreover, a good quality sleep of at least 6 hours every night helps to keep the balance of insulin and blood sugar. Finally, regular checkups help avoid many silent complications of diabetes that show no symptoms.

Regular blood testingto check cholesterol and kidney function will help see problems at the early stages.

VI. THE DIABETIC 2 GROCERY AND FOODS LIST

Food	Measure	Calories	Fat (g)	Fiber (g)	Carbs (g)	Comment
Acesulfame potassium	1/2 gram	0	0	0	0.5	Eat as much as you want
Adzuki beans	1 cup	329	0.5	25	124	**Avoid,** or Limit to 1 cups a day
Agave	1 tbsp	21	0.5	na	76	Eat in moderation (do not exceed 3 times per day)
Aioli	1 tbsp	80	9	0	0	Eat as much as you want
Alfalfa	1 cup	8	0.2	0.6	0.7	Eat as much as you want
Almond butter	1T	98	9g	1.6	3	Eat as much as you want
Almond oil	1T	120	14	0	0	Eat as much as you want
Almonds	1/2 cup	425	38	1.8	13	low in carbs
Apple	1 medium	95	0.3	4.4	25	low in carbs
Apple betty	1 serving	150	4	0.5	29	low in carbs
Apple juice canned	1 cup	125	0	0	34	low in carbs
Apple pie	1 med piece	296	14	2	43	low in carbs
Apple vinegar	1/3 cup	14	0	0	3	Eat as much as you want
Apples, raw	1 med	70	0.3	1	18	low in carbs
Apricots	1 cup	220	0.6	1	57	Eat in moderation (do not exceed 3 times per day)
Artichoke	1 large	Aban-44	0.2	2	10	low in carbs
Arugula (Rocket)	1 leaf	1	0	0 (if one leaf), 1 cup (0.4 g)	0.1	Eat as much as you want
Asparagus	6 spears	18	0	0.5	3	Eat as much as you want
Aspartame	1 tbsp	38.3	0	0	9.4	Eat as much as you want
Aubergine	1 medium	136	1	16	32	low in carbs
Avocado	1/2 large	185	18	1.8	6	Eat as much as you want
Avocado oil	1 tbsp	124	14	0	0	Eat as much as you want
Bacon	2 slices	95	8	0	1	Eat as much as you want
Bagels	1 bagel	245	1.5	4	48	low in carbs
Banana	1 med.	85	0.4	0.9	23	low in carbs
Barley	1 cup	651	4.2	32	135	**Avoid,** or Limit to 1 cups a day

Food	Measure	Calories	Fat (g)	Fiber (g)	Carbs (g)	Comment
Basil	2 tbsp	1	0	0.1	0.1	Eat as much as you want
Bay leaves	1 tbsp	6	0.2	0.5	1.3	Eat as much as you want
Bean soups	1 cup	190	5	0.6	30	low in carbs
Bean sprouts	1 cup	17	0.2	0.3	3	Eat as much as you want
Beans	1 cup	25	2.4	0.8	6	Eat as much as you want
Beans (green)	1 cup	70	0.1	3.4	7	Eat as much as you want
Bearnaise sauce	1 cup	936	**96.9**	na	5.5	Eat as much as you want
Beef	3 oz.	245	16	0	0	Eat as much as you want
Beef soup	1 cup	100	4	0.5	11	low in carbs
Beer	2 cups	228	0	0	8	Eat as much as you want
Beet greens	1 cup	27	0	1.4	6	Eat as much as you want
Beetroots	1 cup	1	0	3.4	0.8	Eat as much as you want
Beets	1 cup	**60**	0.2	3	13	low in carbs
Bell Pepper (Capsicum)	1 cup	31	0	2.5	**5.3**	Eat as much as you want
Biscuits	1	130	4	1.5	18	low in carbs
black pepper	1 teaspoon	7	0.1	0.7	1.9	Eat as much as you want
Blackberries	1 cup	85	1	6.6	19	low in carbs
Blackberry	1 cup	47	0.4	2.9	11	low in carbs
Blueberries	1 cup	245	na	2	65	Eat in moderation (do not exceed 3 times per day)
Blueberry	1 cup	47	0.4	2.9	11	low in carbs
Bok Choy	1 cup	9	0.1	0.7	1.5	Eat as much as you want
Borlotti beans	1 cup	653	2.4	48	117	Limit to 1 cups a day
Bouillon	1 cup	24	0	0	0	Eat as much as you want
Bran flakes	1 cup	117	2.2	0.1	32	low in carbs
Brazil nuts	1/2 cup	457	47	2	7	Eat as much as you want
Brazil nuts	1 oz.	186	19	2	3.5	Eat as much as you want
Bread	1 oz.	75	0.9	0.8	14	low in carbs
Bread pudding	3/4 cup	374	12	0.2	56	Eat in moderation (do not exceed 3 times per day)
Bread, cracked wheat	1 slice	60	1	0.1	12	low in carbs

Food	Measure	Calories	Fat (g)	Fiber (g)	Carbs (g)	Comment
Breakfast cereals	1 cup	307	5	8	55	Eat in moderation (do not exceed 3 times per day)
Broccoli	1 cup	45	0	1.9	8	Eat as much as you want
Brown, firm-packed, dark sugar	1 cup	815	0	0	210	**Avoid**, or do not exceed 1 cup a day, and you should limit your carb intake for the rest of the day to a food that has less than 40g of carbs
Brussels sprouts	1 cup	60	0.3	1.7	12	low in carbs
Butter	1 tbsp	100	11	0	0	Eat as much as you want
Butter	1/2 cup	113	115	117	118	Limit to 1/2 cups a day
Buttermilk	1 cup	127	5	0	13	low in carbs
Cabbage	1 cup	22	0.1	2.2	5	Eat as much as you want
Cabbage Steamed	1 cup	40	**0.32**	1.3	9	Eat as much as you want
Cajun	1 tbsp	5.2	0.2	na	1	Eat as much as you want
Cakes	1 slice	110	0.2	0	23	low in carbs
Candied	1 med.	235	6	1.5	80	Eat in moderation (do not exceed 3 times per day)
Candy	5	104	3	0	19	low in carbs
Cane Syrup	1 tbsp	50	0	0	13	low in carbs
Canned tomatoes	1/2 cup	39	0.3	2.3	9	Eat as much as you want
Cantaloupe	1/2 med.	40	0.5	2.2	9	Eat as much as you want
Cantaloupe/rock melon	1 cup (Diced)	53	0.3	1.4	13	low in carbs
Carbonated drinks Artificially sweetened	12 oz.	0	0	0	0	Eat as much as you want
Carob	2 tbsp	70	3.5	High in fiber	7	Eat as much as you want
Carrots (chopped)	1 cup	45	0.3	0.9	10	low in carbs
Cashews	1/2 cup	392	32	0.9	20	low in carbs
Cauliflower (chopped)	1 cup	30	0.3	1	6	Eat as much as you want
Celeriac	3 1/2 oz.	42	0.3	1.8	9.2	Eat as much as you want
Celery	1 cup	20	0	1	4	Eat as much as you want
Chard steamed	1 cup	30	0.3	1.4	7	Eat as much as you want

Food	Measure	Calories	Fat (g)	Fiber (g)	Carbs (g)	Comment
Cheddar	1-in. cube	70	6	0	0.2	Eat as much as you want
Cheddar, grated cup	1/2 cup	226	19	0	1	Eat as much as you want
Cheese	1 cup	240	11	0	6	Eat as much as you want
Cheese processed	1 oz.	105	9	0	6	Eat as much as you want
Cheese Roquefort type	1 oz.	105	9	0	1	Eat as much as you want
Cherries	1 cup	100	1	2	26	low in carbs
Cherries red	1 cup	77	0.5	2.5	19	low in carbs
Cherries sweet	1 cup	97	0.2	3.2	25	low in carbs
Cherry Pie	1 slice	340	13	0.1	55	Eat in moderation (do not exceed 3 times per day)
Chia seeds	1 oz.	138	9	10	12	low in carbs
chicken	3 oz.	185	9	0	0	Eat as much as you want
Chicken livers, fried	3 med.	140	14	0	2.3	Eat as much as you want
chicken soup	1 cup	75	2	0	10	low in carbs
Chickpeas	1 cup	729	12	35	121	**Avoid,** or,Limit to 1 cups a day
Chicory	1/2 cup	4	0.1	0.8	0.8	Eat as much as you want
Chillies (shopped or diced)	1/2 cup	30	0.3	1.1	7	Eat as much as you want
chinese cabbage	1 cup	9	0.1	0.7	1.5	Eat as much as you want
Chips	1 oz.	152	10	1.4	15	low in carbs
Chives (shopped)	1 tbsp	1	0	0.1	0.1	Eat as much as you want
Chocolate (dark)	1 oz.	155	9	2	17	low in carbs
Chocolate (Milk)	1 oz.	535	30	3.4	59	Eat in moderation (do not exceed 3 times per day)
Chocolate creams	2	130	4	0	24	low in carbs
Chocolate fudge	1 slice	420	14	0.3	70	Eat in moderation (do not exceed 3 times per day)
Chocolate syrup	2 tbsp	80	0.4	0	22	low in carbs
Choy Sum	1 cup	20	0	0	3	Eat as much as you want
Cinnamon	1 tbsp	19	0.1	4.1	6	Eat as much as you want
Clam chowder	1 cup	85	2	0.5	12	low in carbs
Clams	3 oz.	87	1	0	2	Eat as much as you want

Food	Measure	Calories	Fat (g)	Fiber (g)	Carbs (g)	Comment
Clementine	1 medium	35	0.1	1.3	9	Eat as much as you want
Cloves	1 tbsp	18	0.8	2.2	4.3	Eat as much as you want
Club soda	12 oz.	0	0	0	0	Eat as much as you want
Cocoa	1 cup	235	11	0	26	low in carbs
Coconut (shredered)	1 cup	283	27	7	12	low in carbs
Coconut oil	1 tbsp	117	14	0	0	Eat as much as you want
Coconut sugar	1 teaspoon	15	na	na	4	Eat as much as you want
coconut sweetened	1/2 cup	274	20	2	26	low in carbs
Cod	3 1/2 oz.	170	5	0	0	Eat as much as you want
Coffee	1 cup	3	0	0	1	Eat as much as you want
Cola drinks	12 oz.	137	0	0	38	low in carbs
Collard Greens (chopped)	1 cup	11	0.2	1.4	2	Eat as much as you want
Collards (chopped)	1 cup	51	0.2	2	8	Eat as much as you want
Cookies	1 medium cookie	40	1.9	0.1	9	Eat as much as you want
Coriander/cilantro	1 cup	**0.92**	0.02	0.11	**0.15**	Eat as much as you want
Corn	1 ear	92	1	0.8	21	low in carbs
Corn bread ground meal	1 serving	100	4	0.3	15	low in carbs
Corn grits cooked	1 cup	120	1	0.2	27	low in carbs
Corn meal	1 cup	360	4	1.6	74	Eat in moderation (do not exceed 3 times per day)
Corn oil	1 tbsp	125	14	0	0	Eat as much as you want
Corned beef	3 oz.	185	10	0	0	Eat as much as you want
Corned beef hash canned	3 oz.	120	8	**2.34**	6	Eat as much as you want
Corned beef hash Dried	2 oz.	115	4	0	0	Eat as much as you want
Corned beef hash Stew	1 cup	185	10	4.8	15	low in carbs
Cornflakes	1 cup	110	Cornflakes	0.1	25	low in carbs
Cornstarch	1 cup	275	10	0	40	low in carbs
Cottage cheese	4 oz.	111	4.9	0	3.8	Eat as much as you want

Food	Measure	Calories	Fat (g)	Fiber (g)	Carbs (g)	Comment
Couscous	1 oz.	96	0.1	1.2	20	low in carbs
Cows' milk	1 q tbsp	660	40	0	48	low in carbs
Crab meat	3 oz.	90	2	0	1	Eat as much as you want
Crackers	2 med.	55	1	0.2	10	low in carbs
Cranberries	1/3 cup	123	0	2.3	82	Eat in moderation (do not exceed 3 times per day)
Cranberry bean	1 cup	653	2.4	48	117	**Avoid,** or Limit to 1 cups a day
Cranberry sauce sweetened	1 cup	530	0.4	1.2	142	**Avoid,** or Limit to 1 cups a day
Cream	1 cup	315	28	na	9	Eat as much as you want
Cream cheese	1 oz.	105	11	0	1	Eat as much as you want
Cream or half-and-half	1/2 cup	170	15	0	5	Eat as much as you want
Cream soups	1 cup	200	12	1.2	18	low in carbs
Crisps	1 oz.	152	10	1.4	15	low in carbs
Cucumber (chopped)	1 cup	16	0.1	1	3.8	Eat as much as you want
Cucumbers	8	6	0	0.2	1	Eat as much as you want
Cumin	1 teaspoon	0.5	0.5	0.2	0.9	Eat as much as you want
Cupcake	1	160	3	1.8	31	low in carbs
Custard	1 cup	285	14	0	28	low in carbs
Custard dessert	1 slice	265	11	0	34	low in carbs
Daikon	1 medium	61	0.3	5	14	low in carbs
Dandelion greens	1 cup	80	1	3.2	16	low in carbs
Dates	1 cup	505	0.6	3.6	134	Limit to 1/2 cups a day
Donuts (with jelly), donuts with chocolate or with sugar have less carbs, fats, fibers.	1 medium	340	19	0.9	33	low in carbs
Doughnuts	1	135	7	1.3	17	low in carbs
Dried fruit	1 oz.	102	0.8	0	23	low in carbs
Dried, uncooked	1/2 cup	220	t	1	50	Eat in moderation (do not exceed 3 times per day)
Duck (chpped or diced)	1 cup	472	6	0	0	Eat as much as you want
Duck, domestic	3 1/2 oz.	370	28	0	0	Eat as much as you want
Eggplant	1 cup	30	0.1	1	9	Eat as much as you want
Eggplant	1 medium	136	1	16	32	low in carbs

Food	Measure	Calories	Fat (g)	Fiber (g)	Carbs (g)	Comment
Eggs (boiled)	1 large	78	5	0	0.6	Eat as much as you want
Eggs (Omelet)	1 tbsp	23	1.7	0	0.1	Eat as much as you want
Eggs (raw)	1 medium	63	4.2	na	0.3	Eat as much as you want
Eggs raw	2	150	12	0	1.2	Eat as much as you want
Eggs Scrambled or fried	2	220	16	0	1	Eat as much as you want
Endive	1/2 cup	4	0.1	0.8	0.8	Eat as much as you want
Erythritol	4g	1	0	0	4	Eat as much as you want
Evaporated, undiluted	1 cup	345	20	0	24	low in carbs
Farina	1 cup	105	0.9	8	22	low in carbs
Fennel (sliced)	1 cup	27	0.2	2.7	6	Eat as much as you want
Feta	1 oz.	75	6	0	1.2	Eat as much as you want
Figs	2	120	**0.5**	1.9	30	low in carbs
figs Canned with syrup	3	130	na	1	32	low in carbs
Fish	3 oz.	208 (at most)	20 (at most)	0	0	Eat as much as you want
Fish sticks fried	5	200	10	0	8	Eat as much as you want
Flax seeds	1 tbsp	55	4.3	2.8	3	Eat as much as you want
Flounder	3 1/2 oz.	200	8	0	0	Eat as much as you want
Flour	1 cup	460	22	2.9	33	low in carbs
Flour refined	1	115	2	3	20	low in carbs
Fortified milk	6 cups	1,373	42	1.4	119	Limit to 3 cups a day
French dressing	1 tbsp	60	6	0	2	Eat as much as you want
French-fried	10 pieces	155	7	0.4	20	low in carbs
Fresh, raw figs	3 med.	90	0	1	22	low in carbs
Fried, breast or leg and thigh chicken	3 oz.	245	15	0	0	Eat as much as you want
Fruit cake	1 slice	105	4	0.2	17	low in carbs
Fruit cocktail, canned	1 cup	195	0.22	0.5	50	Eat in moderation (do not exceed 3 times per day)
Fruit-flavored soda	12 oz.	161	0	0	42	low in carbs
Fudge	2 pieces	370	12	0.1	80	Eat in moderation (do not exceed 3 times per day)

Food	Measure	Calories	Fat (g)	Fiber (g)	Carbs (g)	Comment
Galangal	1 oz.	20	0	0	4	Eat as much as you want
Game meats	1 oz.	34	0.7	0	0	Eat as much as you want
Garam masala	1/4 teaspoon	1	0	0.1	0.2	Eat as much as you want
Garlic	1 clove	4	0	0.1	0.9	Eat as much as you want
Gelatin, made with water	1 cup	155	0	0	36	low in carbs
Gin	1 oz.	70	0	0	0	Eat as much as you want
Ginger (ground)	1 teaspoon	2	0.1	14	1.3	Eat as much as you want
Ginger ale	12 oz.	105	0	0	28	low in carbs
Gingerbread	1 slice	180	7	0.5	28	low in carbs
Goats' milk	1 cup	165	10	0	11	low in carbs
Granula bar	1 bar	99	4.2	1.1	14	low in carbs
Grape juice	1 cup	160	0.3	0.5	42	low in carbs
Grapefruit	1 cup	97	0.3	3.7	25	low in carbs
Grapefruit, fresh, 5" diameter	2-Farvardin	50	0.2	1	14	low in carbs
Grapes	1 cup	70	0.3	0.8	16	low in carbs
Green beans	1 cup	31	0.1	3.4	7	Eat as much as you want
Ground lean	3 oz.	185	10	0	0	Eat as much as you want
Guacamole	1 tbsp	23	2.08	1	1.24	Eat as much as you want
Guava	1 cup	68	1.6	9	24	low in carbs
Haddock	3 oz.	135	5	0	6	Eat as much as you want
Halibut	3 1/2 oz.	182	8	0	0	Eat as much as you want
Haloumi	1 oz.	110	25	na	1.3	Eat as much as you want
Ham pan-broiled	3 oz.	290	22	0	0	Eat as much as you want
Ham, as	2 oz.	170	13	0	0	Eat as much as you want
Ham, canned, spiced	2 oz.	165	14	0	1	Eat as much as you want
Hamburger	3 oz.	245	17	0	0	Eat as much as you want
Hard candies	1 oz.	90	0	0	28	low in carbs
Hazelnut oil	1 tbsp	120	13.6	0	0	Eat as much as you want
Hazelnuts	1 oz.	178	17	2.7	4.7	Eat as much as you want
Herring	1 small	211	13	0	0	Eat as much as you want

Food	Measure	Calories	Fat (g)	Fiber (g)	Carbs (g)	Comment
Hollandaise sauce	1/2 pack	220	23	0.2	3.9	Eat as much as you want
Honey	2 tbsp	120	0	0	30	low in carbs
Hot sauce.	1 teaspoon	0	0	0	0.1	Eat as much as you want
Hydrogenated cooking fat	1/2 cup	665	100	0	0	Eat as much as you want
Ice cream	2 cups	690	24	0	70	Eat in moderation (do not exceed 3 times per day)
Ice cream	1 cup	300	18	0	29	low in carbs
Ice milk	1 cup	275	10	0	32	low in carbs
Iceberg	1/4 head	13	0.1	0.5	3	Eat as much as you want
Ices	1 cup	117	0	0	48	low in carbs
Jam	1 tbsp	56	0	0.2	14	low in carbs
Jellies	1 tbsp	50	0	0	13	low in carbs
Juice (fruit)	1 cup	136	0	0.5	33	low in carbs
Kale	1 cup	45	1	0.9	8	Eat as much as you want
Kidney beans	1 cup	613	1.5	46	110	**Avoid,** or Limit to 1 cups a day
Kiwi (sliced)	1 cup	110	0.9	5	26	low in carbs
Kohlrabi	1 cup	40	0.1	1.5	9	Eat as much as you want
Kumara (cubes sliced)	1 cup	114	0.1	4	27	low in carbs
Lamb, chop, broiled	4 oz.	480	35	0	0	Eat as much as you want
Lambs quarters, steamed	1 cup	48	1	3.2	7	Eat as much as you want
Lard	1/2 cup	992	110	0	0	Eat as much as you want
Lavender Latte	1/2 teaspoon	16	1	1.2	3.1	Eat as much as you want
Leeks	1 medium	54	0.3	1.6	13	low in carbs
Leg roasted	3 oz.	314	14	0	0	Eat as much as you want
Lemon	1 medium	24	0.3	2.4	8	Eat as much as you want
Lemon grass (citronella)	1 cup	66	0.3	0.4	16.6	low in carbs
lemon juice	1 cup	53	0.2	0.3	17	low in carbs
Lemon meringue	1 slice	300	12	0.1	45	low in carbs
Lemonade concentrate frozen	6-oz. can	430	1.5	0	112	**Avoid** or Limit to 6 oz a day
Lentils	1 cup	212	0.8	2.4	38	low in carbs
Lettuce	1/4 head	14	0.1	0.5	2	Eat as much as you want

Food	Measure	Calories	Fat (g)	Fiber (g)	Carbs (g)	Comment
Lima	1 cup	140	0.7	3	24	low in carbs
Lima, dry, cooked	1 cup	260	**15.7**	2	48	low in carbs
Lime juice	1 cup	60	0.2	1	20	low in carbs
Limeade concentrate frozen	6-oz. can	405	3	0	108	**Avoid,** or Limit to 1 cups a day
Lobster	medium	92	1	0	0	Eat as much as you want
Macadamia nuts	1 oz.	204	21	2.4	3.9	Eat as much as you want
Macaroni	1 cup	155	1	0.1	32	low in carbs
Macaroni Baked with cheese	1 cup	475	25	1	44	low in carbs
Mackerel	3 oz.	155	9	a	0	Eat as much as you want
Mandarin	1 medium	47	0	2.4	12	low in carbs
Mango	1 cup	99	0.6	2.6	25	low in carbs
Maple syrup	1 teaspoon	52	0	0	13	low in carbs
Margarine	1/2 cup	806	91	0	0.8	Eat as much as you want
Margarine	1 tbsp	100	11	0	0.1	Eat as much as you want
Marshmallows	5	98	0	0	23	low in carbs
Mayonnaise	1 tbsp	110	12	0	0.1	Eat as much as you want
Milk 1% fat	1 cup	103	2.4	0	12	low in carbs
Milk 2% fat	1 cup	124	4.9	0	12	low in carbs
Milk 3.7 % fat	1 cup	156	9	0	11	low in carbs
Milk chocolate	2-oz. bar	290	6	0.2	44	low in carbs
Milk non fat	1 cup	83	0.2	0	12	low in carbs
Milk powder	1 cup	635	34	0	49	low in carbs
Milk skim	1 q tbsp	360	na	0	52	Eat in moderation (do not exceed 3 times per day)
Milkshake Chocolat	1 fl Oz	34	0.8	0.1	21	low in carbs
Milkshake Vanilla	1 fl Oz	32	0.9	0	5	Eat as much as you want
Mince	1 slice	340	9	0.7	62	Eat in moderation (do not exceed 3 times per day)
Miso	1 cup	546	17	15	73	Eat in moderation (do not exceed 3 times per day)
Molasses	1 tbsp	45	0	8	11	low in carbs
Monk fruit extract	1 tbsp	0	0	na	0	Eat as much as you want
Muesli bars	1 bar	95	8	4	**32**	low in carbs
Muffins	1	135	5	0.3	19	low in carbs

Food	Measure	Calories	Fat (g)	Fiber (g)	Carbs (g)	Comment
Mung beans	1 cup	718	2.4	34	130	Limit to 1 cups a day
Mushrooms	1 medium	4	0.1	0.2	0.6	Eat as much as you want
Mushrooms canned	4	12	0	2	4	Eat as much as you want
Mustard	1 teaspoon	3	0.2	0.2	0.3	Eat as much as you want
Mustard greens (chopped)	1 cup	30	0.2	1.2	6	Eat as much as you want
Navy beans	1 cup	70	0.7	19	14	low in carbs
Nectarine	1 medium	63	0.5	2.4	15	low in carbs
Noodle	1 cup	115	4	0.2	13	low in carbs
Noodles	1 cup	200	2	0.1	37	low in carbs
Nutella	2 tbsp	200	11	2	23	low in carbs
Nutmeg (ground)	1 tbsp	37	2.5	1.5	3.5	Eat as much as you want
Nuts butter	2 tbsp	188	16	1.9	6	Eat as much as you want
Oatmeal	1 cup	150	3	4.6	26	low in carbs
Oats	1 oz.	120	2.4	3	21	low in carbs
Okra	1 1/3 cups	32	0.2	1	7	Eat as much as you want
Olive oil	1 tbsp	125	14	0	0	Eat as much as you want
Olives (green, black)	1 tbsp	0.9	0.9	0.3	0.5	Eat as much as you want
Olives large	10	72	10	0.8	3	Eat as much as you want
OlivesRipe	10	105	13	1	1	Eat as much as you want
Onions	1	80	0.1	1.6	18	low in carbs
Onions (green) (chopped)	1 cup	32	0.2	2.6	7	Eat as much as you want
or whipping	1/2 cup	430	44	1	3	Eat as much as you want
Orange	1 medium	62	0.2	3.1	15	low in carbs
Orange juice	1 fl oz.	112	0.1	0.2	25	low in carbs
Oregano	1 teaspoon	5.51	0.18	0.77	1.16	Eat as much as you want
Oyster stew	1 cup	125	6	0	0	Eat as much as you want

Food	Measure	Calories	Fat (g)	Fiber (g)	Carbs (g)	Comment
Oysters	6-8 med.	231	233	235	236	**Avoid**, or Do not exceed 8 medium Oysters a day, and you arellowed limit your carb intake for the rest of the day to a food that has less than 20g of carbs
Pancakes 4" diam.	4	250	9	0.1	28	low in carbs
Papaya	1/2 med.	75	0.2	1.8	18	low in carbs
Paprika	1 teaspoon	6	0.3	0.8	1.2	Eat as much as you want
Parsley	2 tbsp	2	0	0.2	0.5	Eat as much as you want
Parsnips	1 cup	95	1	3	22	low in carbs
Passion fruit	1 cup	229	1.7	25	55	Eat in moderation (do not exceed 3 times per day)
Pasta	2 oz	75	0.6	1.8	14	low in carbs
Pastries	1 oz.	156	11	0.4	13	low in carbs
Peaches	1 cup	200	0.2	1	52	Eat in moderation (do not exceed 3 times per day)
Peanut butter	1/3 cup	300	25	0.9	9	Eat as much as you want
Peanut butter, natural	1/3 cup	284	24	0.9	8	Eat as much as you want
Peanuts	1/3 cup	290	25	1.2	9	Eat as much as you want
Pears	1 cup	195	0.2	2	50	Eat in moderation (do not exceed 3 times per day)
Peas	1 cup	66	0.6	0.1	13	low in carbs
Peas (green)	1 cup	118	0.6	7	21	low in carbs
Peas frozen	1 cup		**0.6**	1.8	12	low in carbs
Peas Split cooked	4 cups	115	0.8	0.4	21	low in carbs
Peas, Fresh, steamed	1 cup	70	**0.9**	2.2	12	low in carbs
Peas, heated	1 cup	53	0.22	1	10	low in carbs
Pecans	1/2 cup	343	35	1.1	7	Eat as much as you want
peppermint	2 leaves	0	0	0	0	Eat as much as you want
Peppers with beef and crumbs	1 med.	255	9	1	24	low in carbs
Persimmons	1 med.	75	0.1	2	20	low in carbs
Pesto	1 tbsp	84	8.2	0.2	1.2	Eat as much as you want
Pineapple	1 large slice	95	0.2	0.4	26	low in carbs

Food	Measure	Calories	Fat (g)	Fiber (g)	Carbs (g)	Comment
Pineapple Crushed	1 cup	205	0.2	0.7	55	Eat in moderation (do not exceed 3 times per day)
Pineapple juice	1 cup	120	0.2	0.2	32	low in carbs
Pizza medium	1 section	180	6	17	23	low in carbs
Plain yogurt	1 container	150	11	0	**8**	Eat as much as you want
Plain, with no icing	1 slice	180	5	0.1	31	low in carbs
Plantain	1 medium	57	0.7	4.1	57	Eat in moderation (do not exceed 3 times per day)
Plums (sliced)	1 cup	185	0.5	0.7	50	Eat in moderation (do not exceed 3 times per day)
Pomegranate	1/2 cup	70	1	3	13	low in carbs
Popcorn salted	2 cups	152	7	0.5	20	low in carbs
Pot-pie	1 pie	480	28	3	32	low in carbs
Potato chips	10	110	7	1.4	10	low in carbs
Potatoes Mashed with milk and butter	1 cup	230	12	0.7	28	low in carbs
Potatoes steamed before peeling	1 med.	80	8	0.4	19	low in carbs
Potatoes, pan-tried	3/4 cup	268	14	0.4	33	low in carbs
Potetoes Stewed or canned	1 cup	100	2.5	2	26	low in carbs
Powdered milk	1 cup	515	28	0	39	low in carbs
preserves	1 tbsp	55	0	0.22	14	low in carbs
Pretzels	1 oz.	108	0.7	0.9	23	low in carbs
Prune juice	1 cup	170	0	0.7	45	low in carbs
Prunes	1 cup	300	1	0.8	81	Eat in moderation (do not exceed 3 times per day)
Puddings Sugar	1 cup	770	0	0	199	Do not exceed 1 cup a day,and you are alowed to consume a food that has less than 50 g of carbds for the rest of the day
Puffed rice	1 cup	55	0.1	0.2	12	low in carbs
Puffed wheat presweetened	1 cup	105	0.1	0.6	26	low in carbs

Food	Measure	Calories	Fat (g)	Fiber (g)	Carbs (g)	Comment
Pumpkin Pie	1 slice	265	12	8	34	low in carbs
Pumpkin seeds	1 oz.	126	5	5	15	low in carbs
Quinoa	1 tbsp	14	0.2	0.3	2.5	Eat as much as you want
Radicchio (Shredded)	1 cup	9	0.1	0.4	1.8	Eat as much as you want
Radishes	1 medium	61	0.3	5	14	low in carbs
Radishes	5 small	10	0	0.3	2	Eat as much as you want
Raisins	1/2 cup	230	0.3	0.7	82	Eat in moderation (do not exceed 3 times per day)
Ranch dressing	1 tbsp	73	8	0.1	1	Eat as much as you want
Raspberries Raw	1 cup	54	0.8	1.9	12	low in carbs
Raspberries Raw, diced	1 cup	75	0.8	0.6	19	low in carbs
Raspberries Raw, grated	1 cup	45	0.8	1.2	10	low in carbs
Raspberries Raw, green	6 small	22	0.8	1	5	Eat as much as you want
Raspberries Raw, red	3/4 cup	57	0.8	5	14	low in carbs
Red kidney	1 cup	230	1	2.5	42	low in carbs
Rhubarb sweetened	1 cup	385	0.2	1.9	98	Eat in moderation (do not exceed 3 times per day)
Rice	1 cup	748	3	1.2	154	Do not exceed 1 cup a day
Rice flakes	1 cup	115	1	0.1	26	low in carbs
Rice polish	1/2 cup	132	6	1.2	28	low in carbs
Ricotta	1 cup	428	32	0	7	Eat as much as you want
Roast	3 oz.	305	14	0	0	Eat as much as you want
Roast beef	3 oz.	390	36	0	0	Eat as much as you want
roasted and salted	1/2 cup	439	40	1.8	13	low in carbs
Roasted chicken	3 1/2 oz.	290	20	0	0	Eat as much as you want
Rolls	1 large	411	12	0.1	23	low in carbs
Root beer	12 oz.	140	0	0	35	low in carbs
Rosemary	1 teaspoon	4	0.2	0.5	0.7	Eat as much as you want
Rutabagas	4 cups	32	0	1.4	8	Eat as much as you want
Rye	1 slice	55	1	0.1	12	low in carbs
Saccharin	1 packet	0	0	0	1	Eat as much as you want

Food	Measure	Calories	Fat (g)	Fiber (g)	Carbs (g)	Comment
Safflower seed oil	1 tbsp	125	14	0	0	Eat as much as you want
Sage	1 tbsp	6	0.3	0.8	1.2	Eat as much as you want
Salad dressing	1 tbsp	73	7	0	2.5	Eat as much as you want
Salmon	3 oz.	120	5	0	0	Eat as much as you want
Salsa	100 grams	36	0.2	1.4	0.2	Eat as much as you want
Salt	1 teaspoon	0	0	0	0	Eat as much as you want
Sardines	3 oz.	180	9	0	0	Eat as much as you want
Sauerkraut	1 cup	32	0.3	1.2	7	Eat as much as you want
Scallions	1 medium	5	0	0.4	1.1	Eat as much as you want
Scalloped with cheese potatoes	3/4 cup	145	8	0.4	14	low in carbs
Scallops	3 1/2 oz.	104	8	0	10	low in carbs
Seaweeds	100 grams	306	0.3	306	81	Eat in moderation (do not exceed 3 times per day)
Sesame oil	1 teaspoon	40	4.5	0	0	Eat as much as you want
Sesame seeds	1/2 cup	280	24	3.1	10	low in carbs
Shad	3 oz.	170	10	0	0	Eat as much as you want
Shallot (chopped)	1 tbsp	7	0	0.3	17	low in carbs
Shoulder, braised	3 oz.	285	23	0	0	Eat as much as you want
Shredded wheat biscuit	1	100	1	0.7	23	low in carbs
Shrimp	3 oz.	110	1	0	0	Eat as much as you want
Silverbeet	1 leaf	9	0.1	1.6	1.8	Eat as much as you want
skim, instant	1 1/3 cups	290	0.8	0	42	low in carbs
skim, non-instant	2/3 cup	290	0	1	42	low in carbs
skim. milk	1 cup	128	4	1	13	low in carbs
Snow Peas	1 cup	26	0.1	1.6	**4.8**	Eat as much as you want
Soda, 2 1/2 square	2	45	1	2	8	Eat as much as you want
Sour cream	1 tbsp	23	2.4	0	0.3	Eat as much as you want

Food	Measure	Calories	Fat (g)	Fiber (g)	Carbs (g)	Comment
Soy sauce	1 tbsp	9	0.1	0.1	0.8	Eat as much as you want
Soybeans	1 cup	260	11	3.2	20	low in carbs
Spaghetti with meat sauce	1 cup	285	10	0.5	35	low in carbs
Spanish rice	1 cup	217	4	1.2	40	low in carbs
Spinach	1 cup	26	0	1	3	Eat as much as you want
Split-pea soup	1 cup	147	3	0.5	25	low in carbs
Sponge cake	1 slice	115	2	0	22	low in carbs
Squash	1 cup	35	0.1	0.6	8	Eat as much as you want
Squash winter, mashed	1 cup	95	0.2	2.6	23	low in carbs
Stalk raw	1 large	5	**0.4**	0.3	1	Eat as much as you want
Steak	3 oz.	330	27	0	0	Eat as much as you want
Steak, lean, as round	3 oz.	220	12	0	0	Eat as much as you want
Stevia	serving	0	0	0	0	Eat as much as you want
Strawberries	1 cup	242	0.4	1.3	60	Eat in moderation (do not exceed 3 times per day)
strawberry	1 cup	47	0.4	2.9	11	low in carbs
Strips, from raw	1 mad.	20	13	0.5	5	Eat as much as you want
Sucralose	1 packet	3	0	0	**0.9**	Eat as much as you want
Sugar	1 tbsp	50	0	0	12	low in carbs
Sugar	1 teaspoon	16	0	0	4.2	Eat as much as you want
Sunflower oil	1 tbsp	120	14	0	0	Eat as much as you want
Sunflower seeds	1/2 cup	280	26	1.9	10	low in carbs
Sweet potatoes	1 med.	155	1	1	36	low in carbs
Swiss chard	1 oz.	105	8	0	7	Eat as much as you want
Swordfish	1 steak	180	6	0	0	Eat as much as you want
Syrup	2 tbsp	100	0	0	25	low in carbs
Table (12.2% alcohol)	1/2 cup	100	0	0	5	Eat as much as you want
table blends sugar	2 tbsp	110	0	0	29	low in carbs
Tahini	1 oz.	169	15	2.6	6	Eat as much as you want
Tangerines	I med.	40	0.2	1	10	low in carbs
Tapioca cream pudding	1 cup	335	10	0	42	low in carbs

Food	Measure	Calories	Fat (g)	Fiber (g)	Carbs (g)	Comment
Tarragon (ground)	1 tbsp	14	0.3	0.3	2.4	Eat as much as you want
Tea	1 cup	4	0	0	1	Eat as much as you want
Thousand Island sauce	1 tbsp	75	8	0	1	Eat as much as you want
Thyme	1 teaspoon	1	0	0.1	0.2	Eat as much as you want
Tomato juice	1 cup	50	0.1	0.6	10	low in carbs
Tomato soup	1 cup	175	7	0.5	22	low in carbs
Tomatoes	1 cup	50	3	1	9	Eat as much as you want
Tuna	3 oz.	170	7	0	0	Eat as much as you want
Turkey	3 1/2 oz.	265	15	0	0	Eat as much as you want
Turmeric	1 tbsp	24	**0.31**	**2**	4.4	Eat as much as you want
Turnip greens	1 cup	45	1	1.8	8	Eat as much as you want
Turnips, steamed	1 cup	40	0.1	1.8	9	Eat as much as you want
Vanilla	1 tbsp	38	0	0	1.6	Eat as much as you want
Vanilla extract	1 tbsp	38	0	0	1.6	Eat as much as you want
Veal	3 oz.	185	9	0	0	Eat as much as you want
Vegetable	1 cup	80	2	0	14	low in carbs
Vinaigrette	1 tbsp	72	8	0	0.4	Eat as much as you want
Vinegar	1 tbsp	3	0	0	4.4	Eat as much as you want
Vinegars	1 tbsp	3	0	0	0	Eat as much as you want
Waffles	1	240	9	0.1	30	low in carbs
Walnuts	1/2 cup	325	32	1	8	Eat as much as you want
Watercress stems, raw	1 cup	9	0	0.3	1	Eat as much as you want
Watermelon	1 wedge	120	1	3.6	29	low in carbs
Wheat (all purpose)	1 cup	400	1	0.3	84	Eat in moderation (do not exceed 3 times per day)
Wheat (whole)	1 cup	390	2	2.8	79	Eat in moderation (do not exceed 3 times per day)
Wheat germ	1 cup	245	7	2.5	34	low in carbs
Wheat meal cereal unrefined	3/4 cup	103	1	0.7	25	low in carbs

Food	Measure	Calories	Fat (g)	Fiber (g)	Carbs (g)	Comment
Wheat-germ cereal toasted	1 cup	260	7	2.5	36	low in carbs
Wheat, cooked	3/4 cup	275	1	4.4	35	low in carbs
Wheat, pancakes 4" diam.	4	250	9	0.1	28	low in carbs
Rye, White, 20 slices, or	1-lb. loaf	1,225	15	9	229	**Avoid**, Do not exceed 1 lb. loafs a day, and you should to limit your carb intake for the rest of the day to a food that has less than 20g of carbs
Whole-wheat	1 slice	55	1	0.31	11	low in carbs
whole-wheat	1	102	1	0.1	20	low in carbs
Wines	1/2 cup	164	0	0	9	Eat as much as you want
Winter squash (cubes)	1 cup	40	0.2	1.7	10	low in carbs
with tomatoes and cheese	1 cup	210	5	0.5	36	low in carbs
Yams (cubes)	1 cup	177	0.3	4	27	low in carbs
Yellow Summer Squash (sliced)	1 cup	18	0.2	1.2	3.79	Eat as much as you want
Yolks	1 Large	55	4.5	0	0.6	Eat as much as you want
Zucchini (Courgette) (Chopped)	1 cup	21	0.4	1.2	3.9	Eat as much as you want

end !